Care Giving Gift
of
UNCONDITIONAL
LOVE

DAVID SOH POH HUAT

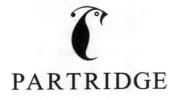

PARTRIDGE

To order additional copies of this book, contact
Toll Free +65 3165 7531 (Singapore)
Toll Free +60 3 3099 4412 (Malaysia)
orders.singapore@partridgepublishing.com

www.partridgepublishing.com/singapore

CONTENTS

DEDICATION

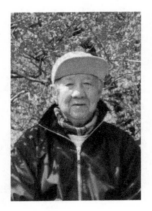

This book is dedicated to my late father
Thomas Soh Yew Chong who passed away
on August 21st, 2011 from Pneumonia.
I would also like to dedicate this to the United
Arab Emirates' families whom I have met whilst
their families sought medical treatment in
Singapore and to their departed loved ones.

DISCLAIMER

This book is written based on observation
and personal experiences
with no intention to offend anyone personally.

Hopefully this book will serve its purpose
to Caregivers and their Families.

PREFACE

Firstly, I would like to thank Our

Lord and Mother Mary

for inspiring me to write this book.

Caregiving to me is a calling

and when one is called,

she or he has to give unconditional love

from their heart, not their mind.

Like our Blessed Mother Mary,

the moment she discovered her

cousin Elizabeth was pregnant

she just leaves everything at home

and went to visit her.

Based on observations and experiences,

many thought that caregiving is just providing

the 'financial' and nothing more.

They forgot that the gift from the

HEART unconditionally

is more important.

Hopefully, this book will 'open

reader's eyes' just like

when 'Thomas eyes were opened

when he met JESUS'

Last but not least, my beloved wife Catherine;

who gives me endearing moral support all the

way and helping me in editing this book to

be an impactful and inspiring piece of art.

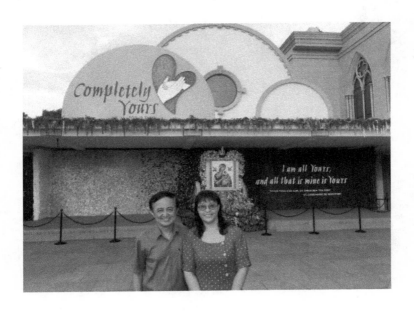

ACKNOWLEDGEMENT

I would like to thank the staff of Partridge Publishing Singapore especially Ms Kathy Lorenzo Publishing Consultant, Senior Publishing Consultant Ms Jade Bailey and Mr Eugene Hopkins for assisting me in making this book possible.

THE STORY BEGINS

With the background of my late father, late sister, and as well as experiences gained from my United Arab Emirates friends who came to Singapore to seek Medical Treatment.

Late Father Thomas Soh Yew Chong

My late father retired when the British Royal Air Force (RAF) withdrew their forces from Singapore in 1968.

After his retirement, he continued to have an active lifestyle meeting friends and travelling overseas with them.

Unfortunately, in 2006, he had a fall which changed his lifestyle and needed to be on a wheelchair. Despite being on a wheelchair, we managed to travel with him to Hainan and Beijing.

In June 2011, his condition worsens and he passed away on 21, August 2011 from Pneumonia.

After his passing, the experience gained as a caregiver always prompted me to ask myself "why I did not do this or that?"

I always believe that this experience has a reason and purpose in one's life and that is what I want to share in this book.

Late Sister Susan Soh Sung Choo

My late sister was with Singapore Airlines Limited. She had Ovarian Cancer in 2005 and undergone chemotherapy after her operation.

From 2005 after her recovery, she was very cautious with her food and ensured that the food taken are organic, no raw or barbequed food etc. She even travelled regularly with my mother and late father.

Yearly, the doctor would schedule a CT scan for her until year 2014, where no scan was scheduled before her yearly visit to the Doctor. Her cancer apparently relapsed.

She subsequently needed to undergo another surgery and Chemotherapy.

After her operation, the Oncologist said that there were still cancer cells and needs Chemotherapy. Her surgeon who is an Associate Professor was surprised and she together with her assistant Doctor confirmed that there were no Cancer cells present. From this experience, we decided to seek Private Oncologists for her subsequent treatments.

From end 2015, she underwent treatments with the Private Oncologists and survived till 3, Nov 2020 when she passed away as the Clear Cells Cancer has infected her lungs.

The last five years journey has gained me bountiful experiences which will be shared in subsequent chapters.

United Arab Emirates Patients seeking medical treatment in Singapore

One of my business is providing accommodation for United Arab Emirates (UAE) citizens coming to Singapore for medical treatment. This business started in 2016.

Based on my late father's and sister's experiences, I have a passion to share my experiences with the patients from UAE.

They have trust and faith in our medical system, but as we know in this world, no one is PERFECT, not even me and only GOD is perfect.

That is why I am also dedicating this book to their families as we became good friends. Some of their loved ones has also passed on.

The experiences gained are invaluable.

REQUIREMENTS

There are many and I will share a few key areas based on observations and experiences.

Family Members as Caregivers

Normally, when a loved one is sick, these are the four likely situations a family will face:

- Siblings will try to avoid taking the lead to care for their loved ones as they are afraid to give financial support. Most cases will fall on one family member.

- Siblings will not care as they are already married out and no longer hold the paternal surname. Well, for me, such siblings should not even exist as it reflects their own family and partner's mental instability.

- Siblings who know that their loved ones have no wealth to leave behind they do not bother to care.

- Siblings only show care for loved ones who have wealth hoping to gain the wealth when they passed away.

The above scenarios are real in this materialistic world of ours and that is why for Caregiving, it has to be totally UNCONDITIONAL and must come from the HEART and not the MIND.

Caregiving is a VOCATION and not everyone has this gift, people who are able to see whether the person is genuine.

Employing Foreign Domestic Workers and Caregivers

This is a real challenge and like "roulette", there is no you can get a perfect one in this world.

How do we ensure it's the right person to employ?

Here are some pointers which is not exhaustive.

- List your own requirements like nationality, age, marital status, their family and experience.

- Can they cook and do housework? Needs to be specific as some will say they are employed as caregiver and should not do housework.

- Type of care required for family member i.e., elderly or sick and type of sickness.

- Past work experiences, if possible, get testimonials.

These are some of the salient points.

UNDERSTANDING THE SITUATION

By staying positive: How?

We need to be in control of the situation when we ourselves as caregivers or our loved ones consult a medical practitioner (doctor).

Diagnosis

When we go for consultation, do have an objective mindset.

To find out what is the result of the tests and any treatment available.

The doctor after analyzing the medical reports will normally give his views and recommendations and what further tests to confirm the findings.

Most of the time, the patient will be shocked with the results and does not know what to do except to listen to the doctor.

The doctor may or may not be top specialists in the country, so we as patients need to be fully aware of what treatment will be given and do our own personal research.

We need to bear in mind that in this real world of ours that no one is perfect.

Questions to ask the Doctor either by the patient or caregiver:

- Treatment plan, duration, type of treatment, costs etc.

- What is the likely cause of the illness?

- Will the treatment cure the illness?

- Any other alternatives

- Request for a copy of all the reports

Let the doctor knows you will think about it and discuss with family members.

Seeking second or third opinion

The role of the caregiver is very important at this juncture as the patient will be trying to accept the diagnosis.

Remember that if the caregiver is one who care from the heart, he or she will need to commit totally to ensure that the patient will have the best.

The caregiver and patient should adopt the **5 C's**:

- **C**heck the internet to understand more about the illness.

- **C**heck with other specialists for a second or third opinion.

- **C**heck if the first treatment plan recommended is feasible or is there other alternatives.

- **C**heck if there are trial drugs available.

- **C**aregiver should compile the recommendations and discuss with family members for decision.

Let's ask ourselves, who is more qualified to follow the patient during consulting or treatment? Is it their family member or their foreign domestic workers or not related caregiver?

Some family members will do otherwise which is very sad.

Hopefully, these real-life cases will be beneficial to all.

Palliative Care

There will come a time when our loved ones are in the Final Stage of their life and we need to ask ourselves

1. Should we send them to a HOSPICE for their palliative care and let them passed on without their loved ones around.

Or

2. Should we let them stay at home with their loved ones and create conducive environment

for them like having standby medical equipment, hospital bed etc.

We may even need to engage 24 hour nursing service to look after them as the employed caregiver is no longer qualified or competent to look after our loved ones.

As there are many 24 hours Nursing Services available, we need to know our needs for our sick loved ones prior to engaging them.

Understanding the STAFF below:

i. Staff qualifications – experienced or trainee nurses.

ii. Their skills in taking care of elderly or cancer patients.

iii. Any experience in doing blood test or handling medical equipment.

iv. Fixed nurses throughout the period.

v. Find out the costs of various providers available.

We need to be in control again as some of these providers will just provide the service as a business and will lack the personal care and attention.

TRUSTING AND MOVING FORWARD

Many did not realize the role of the **CAREGIVER** is very important, just like a Pregnant Mother carrying the fetus in her womb for nine months.

Some family members will just leave everything to the foreign domestic worker or employed caregiver without realizing the importance of family care.

As my late father caregiver, Pneumonia is unknown to me until after my father passed away that is when I discovered the causes.

Caregivers, please do not be complacent and treat Pneumonia as nothing.

Will be sharing more real-life cases and let readers be aware what is happening in this real world.

LIFE EXPERIENCE

PNEUMONIA

Pneumonia is the number 1 killer for elderly in some countries. Are we going to accept it and do nothing or we do preventive measures?

Some family members will just ignore and treat it as a part of the aging process which is ridiculous.

I am sharing this based on my late father's experience.

Are we aware that there are two tubes from our mouth, one, the Trachea leads to our left and right lung for breathing? One, the Esophagus leads to the stomach for food digestion. This shows how complex our body is. We have a great creator.

Symptoms

When one tend to cough or choke frequently whenever he or she is eating or drinking these are possible symptoms.

Possible cause

What exactly happens is that the food and drink is supposed to flow through the Esophagus tube to the stomach but instead, the Trachea tube does not close properly thus allowing some food and water to slip through and enter the lung. As we age, the muscles do not react fast enough to close.

What's next?

The foreign food particles and water which enter the lung over time will infect the lung as more water enters the Pneumonia kicks in. The person will have signs of body weakness and fever.

Preventive action

Well, if the cough and choke tend to be frequent, request the doctor to refer to the Speech Therapist. Most will not refer and say it is common for elderly, do insist.

Speech Therapist

They will assess the person swallowing pattern and the two tubes functionality and advise what to do.

Testimonials

A friend needs to be on tube feeding because of Pneumonia. After suggesting to her to see the speech therapist, Praised the Lord and with her Faith as well, she eats and do not need to use the tube feeding but must do some action before swallowing.

Why I share this? Some caregivers will just accept this as part of growing old and just do nothing.

LIVER ABSCESS

My late father at age 87 was diagnosed of liver abscess and the doctor scheduled him to undergone chemotherapy.

Fortunately, a friend recommended us to seek a second opinion from a private liver specialist. This doctor specialized in Radio Frequency Ablation (RFA) which during that time there are not many such specialist around. My father opted for this treatment instead of Chemotherapy which does less damage to his health than the latter. After his treatment, within a month we travelled for a short vacation.

Can we imagine if the caregiver does not explore other alternatives, what will happen to the patient under their care?

CANCER

If a patient has been treated by the doctor and recovered but the Cancer relapsed after ten years what should the caregiver or patient do?

Be complacent and continue to trust the same doctor or have an analytical mind and explore other alternatives.

Most caregivers and patients will just continue with the same doctor thinking that the doctor has been treating the patient for a long time and it is better to remain as it is.

Many caregivers and patients failed to understand sometimes these doctors are

- Complacent and does not explore alternative treatment

- Arrogant so caregivers and patients are scared to question the doctor to clarify the relapse.

- Not caring as they do not see any hope the Cancer patient recovery.

Like my late sister case in 2015, her doctor only gave her about one year of life span.

As her caregiver and having discussed with her, we seek treatment in a Private Clinic and she survived five more fruitful years.

During the five years, her doctor was excellent as she was able to engage with the patient and caregivers constructively and willing to explore any alternative treatment.

Sometimes, caregivers need to think out of the box and do their research for the patient needs and medical treatment and not be too complacent.

We need to remember even Doctors are not perfect as they are human and have their flaws as well.

MR. MOHAMMED (Age 40) seeking treatment in Singapore

Mr. Mohammed was in Singapore for treatment. He knows his illness and I suggested to him to "test" the doctor competency by letting the doctor gives his findings through a translator although he understands English.

To his surprise, after the translation to his native language, the diagnosis was totally different from what the doctor said. With the result he seeks a second opinion for his treatment.

This is sad but is a fact of life.

MRS. TAN (Age 45) had her Tumor removed

Mrs. Tan has a successful surgery but the doctor still recommended her for chemotherapy. She wanted to do a PET scan to check if there are any more tumors but due to hospital procedure, the doctor refused to do it for her.

She subsequently went for a PET scan at a private clinic which confirmed that all are cleared and she therefore did not proceed with the Chemotherapy.

Imagine the above cases, the role of the caregiver is very important as the life of the patient is under their care.

MRS. KHALED (Age 35)

An oversea family shared about wife's Cancer treatment and how they have lost confidence with her doctor as they do not see much progress. They assume that they have the best doctor to give them the treatment but they forgot that sometimes they are not getting the best.

Based on my experience, what they are lack of is a good caregiver as they put their total trust in the system.

I subsequently advised them to seek a second opinion which they did but the system does not permit them to change their doctor.

Much can be done, but sad to say their loved ones passed on in their country.

MR. AHMAD (Age 38)

The patient has been undergoing treatment for the past year at a private clinic. Since their accommodation is under my care, I will always inquire about their condition and showed concern.

Suggested to him to inquire for a second opinion and whether there are 'trial drugs'.

After the patient went for a second opinion and returned to his original clinic, the patient was surprised that the treatment given was changed as well as the medication.

Can we imagine if the patient did not seek a second opinion, he will probably be having the same treatment and medication for a long time.

The patient was subsequently discharged, returned to his country but passed away a few months later.

Such encounter was very sad, if only they have caregivers who are able to guide them along.

MISS TOH (Age 58)

The family employed a foreign domestic worker cum caregiver to look after an elderly and a sick family member.

The family member not staying with them, pays the foreign domestic worker salary and just leave it to her to manage to the elderly and sick to manage.

Is this right or wrong?

- House cleanliness not maintained.

- Meals mostly include instant cereal meals or food ordered from hawker or restaurant. In the long term, these may not be healthy.

- Does not observe any difference or changes in daily behavior and take it as normal.

Advice to all who does such practice, please manage and make sure the caregiver does the right thing. I am sure there are many situations and some family members does not bother as they will just pay their salaries and has no personal commitment to ensure that things are done right.

Bear in mind that caregiving is a Vocation from the Heart and not Mind. By just paying the salary and do not bother, might as well do not do it.

MADAM ALICE (Age 87)

Madam Alice family lets the foreign domestic worker (caregiver) accompany her to the doctor.

My personal thought the family members should accompany and not leave it to them. Why?

- Will the doctor tell the non-family member everything?

- Will the non-family member ask the doctor the right questions?

For example if a doctor gives a prescription for the patient and another doctor advised not to take, who should they believe?

If the family member is in control, then he or she will be able to ask the doctor why it should not be taken.

As a person age, common illness like cataract or dementia will occur. A good caregiver should be proactive and asked the doctor what to look out for and any symptoms to note.

Caregivers should always ask the doctor about regular full blood tests especially for elderly. These are necessary to know the patient's health conditions.

We must always remember, employed caregiver or foreign domestic worker treatment of the elderly or sick differs a lot from their own family members love and care.

MISS JOANNA (Age 38)

Miss Joanna was diagnosed with stage 4 Cancer. Family members and close friends would sometimes try to show their care and concern by recommending health supplements to her without doing further research.

Though their intentions are good, they did not realize that it may do more harm than good.

Miss Joanna was given a supplement by her sister which is supposed to treat her Cancer, but unknowingly, she was unaware that it has a component which is an "energy booster" and can increase the growth of the Cancer cells.

Sometimes the caregiver and patient need to do their own research before consuming.

MRS. FATIMAH (Age 48)

The patient completed her surgery which involved removing tumor around her breast. Patient and daughter were confused during subsequent checkup when the doctor informed them that there were still some tumors.

Having shared with me the diagnosis, I advised them in the capacity of a friend and 'caregiver', that they should seek a second opinion as it is could mean that the doctor may not have done a good job.

They did and subsequently were informed that no further surgery is required.

What if they did not seek second opinion? Caregivers should take note of this.

MISS MAGGIE (Age 42)

Miss Maggie was supposed to consume some health supplements daily at a specific time. Instruction was given to the foreign domestic worker (caregiver).

Apparently, the foreign domestic worker (caregiver) failed to do so.

With no proper supervision by a family member caregiver, the foreign domestic worker (caregiver) failed in her duty and this also applies to the family member for being ignorant in her supervision.

This is really sad as in the end it is the elderly and the sick who suffers and not the caregiver or employer.

We need to ask ourselves, are there any Care and Concern given by the employer by so called leaving everything to the employed caregiver?

We need to remember that what the sick and the elderly need are their own family member care and commitment and not just an employed caregiver.

HOME TO OUR CREATOR

Yes, our time on earth is in HIS TIME.

If the patient had recovered, every day onwards is considered as "bonus" time.

How many family caregivers would be able to say this?

When their loved ones had passed away, I have done my best for them.

For some family members who will only visit the sick when they are hospitalized or when they passed away, how this reflects their filial piety.

There are those who will show their character when their member passed away and their only concern is on the deceased wealth.

Caring for LOVED ONES when they are still alive is a challenge for CAREGIVERS who truly give from their HEARTS as Caregiving is a Vocation and Calling from the HEART and not MIND.

What is the use of offering prayers for their souls after they have passed away rather than caring for them when they are alive?

The Greatest Gift

of all is to treasure

the Memories we had

with our departed loved ones.

-David Soh

ABOUT THE AUTHOR

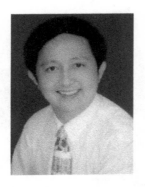

With the successful launched of my first
book **"NATURE GIFTS OF THE SOURSOP
LEAVES"**, it prompted me to write this second
book which I personally felt **CAREGIVING**
has to be from the **HEART** unconditionally.
During my journey as a caregiver for me
late father THOMAS SOH YEW CHONG,

I have discovered a lot of things which
patient and caregivers are fearful to ask.
Likewise, my late sister's journey was an experience
which made me want to really reach out to
people and let them know that there is HOPE
and have FAITH in their recovery process.

Thank you and GOD BLESS